Thera-Diet

The program that incorporates Eating training to promote change in a person's unhealthy eating behavior.

This program can successful when used alone or it can be a supplement with most weight loss diets.

This plan addresses the actual behavior of eating, reframing thought and addressing emotional needs with successful training of eating behavior.

Table of Contents

Forward

This book is written for the following people. The overweight, the obesity, lap band and Bariatric surgery recipients. The program is not a diet. It is an empowering change in ones awareness of self-defeating eating rituals. This program deals with where real change happens; the mind, and its powerful belief systems, motivation and behaviors. The program is written by a therapist that is sympathetic and understands battling weight issues, not a so-called "Gym Rat". A "Gym Rat" is someone that has never been over-weight in their entire life. Then they happen to pursue life as fitness trainers. They may be able to design fitness programs and tell people how they should eat to lose weight, but remember most of them have never experienced doing their so-called weight loss programs as a person of size. Generally they have always had that fast metabolism that supports their perfect model physical appearance. I personally have weighed 330 pounds and had gone on a diet a with exercise program and lost down to 175 pounds. I bulked up with the body builders only to quit the program and regain most of my weight. After implementing this eating behavioral training program for 3 months I was able to lose down to 240 pounds without exercise. Now that I exercise, I'm continuing to shape up my body and feel fabulous. I now experience the association of a positive mental fulfillment feeling with my new developed lifestyle of staying healthy. Believe me, this feeling is contagious in other aspects of my life. As now upon eating a orange, I know the nutrients are assisting my body and I imagine how this fruit that taste so good (stimulating a positive emotion of doing well in taking care of my body) is a healthy way to snack. Learning the techniques of the program and applying them can help you retrain your eating behaviors. This retraining happens in the mind and is carried out with behavioral responses. Through a person's production of experiential awareness, their motivation improves and they continue the management of eating behavioral training. This desire increases ones internal thoughts in reprogramming a positive self belief system about one's self worth and image.

One day as I approached one of those Gym Rats who owned a health club and attempted to work out a deal for a 6 week program for my clients that signed up for my program. An Aura of negativity started saturating during our conversation. His body seemed to communicate a disapproval message when he forcefully engaged his knowledge of weight loss. He Asked, "why I wasn't coming into his Gym and working out?" His attitude projected an interpretation expressing, what I was doing wasn't working. I then countered with confrontational information that I have just lost over 40 pounds in 3 months. I sensed he never really understood because he was one of the Gym Rats that never experienced being over- weight. Of course He did remark that I could gain some muscle and still lose more fat on his program. I didn't argue as he could of never accepted it. After all, I bet I lost more weight and clothes size in the last three months than he ever has in his entire life. This is where I became aware that this is not the place for my clients.

This is a place where their value system is valued on who can become the fittest or build the best body. Usually, my clients are very over weight and don't need another negative person to devalue their accomplishments. No one would ever win in this type of race. I'm not saying all trainers are Gym rats. There are some excellent trainers that can teach me and others some valuable techniques and have a client centered attitude.

Understand that people do not consciously choose to become overweight; it is a consequence of unhealthy patternmatic self harming thinking, learned behavioral habits, and coping skill adaptation. The conscious choice is the selection of foods pairing with the trained eating

4

behavioral rituals. This is a powerful program that will assist you in dramatically changing your life, starting with your mind. Someday you may even become one of those people with that fabulous perfect body. Success is possible if you are willing to face your internal self defeating thoughts, and challenge yourself to step out of a self-imposed comfort zone. Fears of change only reinforce the mental prison. You have to ask yourself "Am I ready and willing to start living once again by facing myself?" If you gave an honest answer of yes, then you are meant to purchase this program. I believe things happen for a purpose and something inspired you to read this book. Think about it. This is the program that you have been looking for. As a bonus, the author has designed a downloadable hypnotic audio script to assist you in achieving your weight loss goals. In order to receive this program, you must visit my website and enter information and proof of purchase. The process will only take a minute or two and the unlocking code or downloadable attachment will be emailed to you. You can contact me personally through my website. I enjoy personally responding to customer emails.

Joseph D. Hayes MS,LPC,NCC. has a website to where he has designed many other self help products. Go to www.coolanger.com to contact, view or sign up for his free news letter.

Acknowledgements

I would like to thank the following people for their contributions to the book and in my life.

Deborah Chelette Wilson MHR.: Who helped me accept that accomplishments are possible through hard work. Deborah has authored an excellent book.

Debra Williamson MS.: Whom I wish all school counselors were as knowledgeable in working with children. I anxiously wait her getting her practicing licensing and going into private practice.

Rhonda Hollins BS.: For her continued patience in helping me with my writing, and especially editing of this book.

Dylan Hayes: My oldest son that assisted in all designing and formatting of the book. He had demonstrated the marvelous ability of biting his tongue in essence of my frantic interaction in designing the cover. Plus upon his birth, I was blessed through God with the meaning and purpose in life.

Thomas Hayes: My youngest son for putting up with my frantic moments during creating the book. He proved to me that the parent curse does exist. Now I apologize to my Family for the moments of dealing with me in my upbringing. By the way, "the curse does work" Thomas.

 Thomas Seaborne PhD.: A remarkable person that is a true inspiration to any person. I am honored to have taken Karate under such a legend. Dr. Seabourne has authored several books in his field of Health/Fitness and knowledge of Sports Psychology.

<u>My Dysfunctional family</u>: Whom I do love and care for very much. Thanks for if I have had a chance to choose to be born again under any family, I would pick the exact same one. They helped me grow and developed who I am today.

<u>My friend Johnny Fulce:</u> Who has been a good friend during times of need. Good luck, I am proud of your song that is being produced. I think it sounds great.

<u>Curt Pitton M.A.</u>: A brilliant therapist, supervisor and good friend. Thank you for allowing me the opportunity to learn and grow as a therapist & person.

Thera-Diet: Eating Behavioral Training

Everyone today is advertising their magic pill or as some would call them snake oil diets and products. It is hard to decipher what will help and what is just a hoax. This material will, hopefully, help you lose weight and start a new life. There are some people that are so far gone that they would need a team of professionals to aid their recovery. This is not written for them. This is for the person of size who is still able to do some physical exercise combined with some healthy behavioral changes. I always say consult your physician before starting any diet/weight loss program. However, this program does not recommend diets. It deals with the true source of the problem, your internal self. I will include: Imagery, a self-empowering motivational hypnotic CD, and challenging thought replacement to assist you in discovering the new transformation that is inside of you and screaming to get out. It is time to wake up and smell the coffee. You have the power to change the way you think, behave, feel and act. Internalizing the things that I am going to teach you, will dramatically increase your self-worth, confidence and just flat out make you feel proud of yourself and your body. Take it from me; I too have been the victim of living too comfortably and allowing myself to become fat. Actually, most of my life has been a battle of the bulge. Now, I accept responsibility and the initiative to take charge of my life. So, if you think it takes expensive gym memberships or gadgets to become fit, you are wrong. I personally would spend my money on a high, quality pair of running shoes. Believe me. You will get your money's worth with the shoes. The gadgets usually become just a good place to hang your ironing.

The reason most of us get fat is we become too comfortable in our sedentary life. One must accept that he/she is self-sabotaging oneself with self-defeating thoughts and habitual, unhealthy behaviors. Sure there are some genetics involved, but without the environmental catalyst they can remain dormant. Genetics are like a light switch. It is hard wired to produce light or allow darkness. Even with the hardwire structure; it takes an action from the environment to be turned on. Maybe I am going a little far with this nature vs. nurture; after all, it has been an age old debate. I just believe that the majority of overweight people are not realizing their true genetic potential. Then they reinforce the overweight situation with the internalized self-defeating thought of "the reason I'm fat is because of genetics." These internal thoughts are also called belief systems and they are nothing more than the way we talk to ourselves. So imagine talking to yourself in this manner. Surely the behavior would create a self-fulfilling prophecy. We are creatures of habit and comfort. Negativity is contagious to all parts of our thinking. One negative thought leads to another. Before long one has created a highway of negativism. In psychology, this would constitute the depressive thinking activity in the back of the brain. After all, each thought is nothing more than neuronal firing; therefore the brain's activity in a depressed person is more active in the back of the brain instead of the front. This is why, I believe, we still have tremendous power within our genetic capabilities to change our lives for the better. I believe there is a positive correlation between depression and overweight people. People become slaves to habit. They go to work and look forward to their lunch break. Wow! What a coincidence. Now a person is set up by his environment to feel good about taking a break and eating at the same time. This would grow into what I call eating pleasure. Pavlov called it a conditioned response. Watson called it reinforcement. Whomever you like, they all have the same thing in common: a pairing of either enjoyment or relaxation with the behavior of eating. There are so many examples, such as celebrating holidays with eating, I can give you, but I will remain on subject. Now, when we feel depressed, bored or nervous, the habitual response is to eat something. We do it so much it becomes almost an unconscious routine behavior. I myself remember eating a whole bucket of popcorn, while watching a movie only to believe I was hungry again 30 minutes later because I saw it was lunch time. See how much impact our thinking has on our physiological bodies. The mind tells the body it is 12 o'clock so it must be time to eat. The body responds with a conditioned response and we behaviorally act out in habit or comfort. This becomes routine and compounds the internal self-defeating thought of "I am just fat because of genetics, so I may as well enjoy myself when I eat".

An unawareness that many overweight people endure right now at this very moment in life is the fact that they are trapped in their own thoughts and behaviors. Awareness is necessary for change. I believe if these people were truly honest with themselves, they would proclaim they are miserable. They have just grown so use to life being a certain way, they have internalized these beliefs and are unfortunately living them out. Change is scary. So, why not battle the monster they are familiar with? The other one is unknown.

I believe people change for three reasons. The first reason is that they are healthy and want to continue a healthy direction in their lives. This would be the people who take yoga to improve their life, not because they are stressed out. That is nice if you happen to be one of those people, but most people I see change out of frustration. They are sick and tired of living life the way they have been. Sometimes these people have hit rock bottom. You see this change in drug addiction recovery. People use the fuel of anger, hurt or fear to motivate a behavioral change. The third reason people change is what I call an existential meaning change. This is when something greater than us happens and we change our lives. An example is having a heart attack and recovering only then to start living a life of healthy eating and exercising. Another example is when a loved one dies; it impacts us so deeply we react with a change in our lives. This changing event usually consists of a divine intervention that I contribute to God. No, you do not have to buy into this last reason to lose weight, nor do you have to believe in God for this program to work. This just is a personal belief of mine. Whichever reason is the catalyst to your change, there is no time like the present to start.

The Here and Now (present) is the most important segment of time in a weight loss program. This is the moment you will endure all challenges of eating decisions, exercising and behaviors. To quote the NIKE logo, "just do it" sums it all up. No excuses. It is time to work and do the weight loss program. I often hear people tell me that they tried a program without success and whine about how they are doomed. The type of mind set you need is **trier's are liars then criers that end up becoming rationalizer's.** Once again, in order to break bad habits it takes a strong behavioral intervention. For example, while in line at a fast food restaurant your thoughts probably go like "Hmm. The double meat hamburger with curly fries sounds good". Then you behave with ordering that exact selection of food. You need to think "I will have the grilled chicken on wheat with fruit. This is a healthy selection" and then just order that way. The self-defeating thoughts are going to haunt you with "You could have had a good tasting meal instead of that unflavored healthy one. I really am suffering on this program" See how the mind turns against you. I do not personally know too many overweight people who have suffered except by their own thoughts. I look at reality and point out that suffering is happening in Ethiopia. So please by all means explain to me how your suffering is similar. Another reframing belief is that I now must eat healthy due to all the previous overindulgence I have had. The important part is to become aware of the internalized eating thought.

11

"eating for pleasure" and reframe that to "I need to eat for healthy nourishment". All this happens internally in the Here and Now and that is where you will face all challenges. These challenges can be won simply by ordering the healthy choice food and just working out. You will be challenged by self-defeating thoughts concerning not doing any physical activity. Just do it and feel better about yourself, because there are thousands of excuses you can choose from to justify not exercising. You can always go back to your old behaviors if you desire. However, you know doing something over and over again and expecting a different result is pure insanity.

People can be Negative

Now that you have made the decision to get healthy and in shape, I would like you to understand behavioral put downs from others. Other people will bombard you with negativity about the way you are doing the program, or how you are not making progress. These people have general negative concepts and tend to look at others and magnify any possible negative point about that person. These people can not stand to look at themselves. Their lives are full of misery. They tend to have a distorted thinking that if I put down others, I look better to myself (or feel better about myself) or they feel like they are important by pointing out negative points. They become empowered by seeing others disappointment. They are unhealthy and can be dealt with by a favorite phrase of mine. "That's very unfortunate" or "I'm on top of that". Notice there seems to be some sort of validation with these phrases; however, I never agreed nor changed my thinking to theirs. See they just bought into the idea that I agreed with them. This is important because one probably would not gain anything by engaging them. These people will shut up when they feel empowered through validation. Unfortunately, they need to see people in turmoil to get this validation. A person on a weight loss program needs to develop coping skills to deal with these types of people. They also can seek out people who are supportive in nature. Sometimes one becomes aware of draining relationships and terminates them. I have seen this in my experience. They tend to be happier and successful after ridding their life of negativity. Do not get me wrong and think you have to get a divorce because your spouse is one of these negative people. Just be aware that many changes will come with your new life of weight loss.

Changing your appearance will affect your life in many ways. One can expect to be treated differently by the opposite sex in public. My own experiences have reinforced this differential treatment. I have experienced more flirtatious behaviors from the opposite sex. I lost a lot of weight after my divorce in 1998. I buffed up and exercised all the time. One day I went into Pizza Hut and ordered a pizza. When it was done, the lady smiled and said, "It's on the house." I was stunned because during my last four fat years, I ordered and ate thousands of pizza and not once had this happened. Once I was even made to dig in my car's ashtray for twenty-five cents. Many entitlements were given to me by overfriendly females. Another thing that I experienced was women making eye contact and smiling or staring. When I was fat, they looked down as if I did not exist or gave me a look of disgust. I remember studies showing that people were rated more attractive when they were fit than when they were overweight. Common sense tells us that the more attractive a person appears; the more opportunities or favors are presented to them. Other things that are positive are more ease in finding a variety of better fitting clothing, and more comfort and better fit public seating. The flip side is usually the change of one's playgrounds and playmates. You will buy clothes that fit and may change your values in clothes. They fall in love with self and tend to change associations with others. Now a physical body change heavily influences the inner-self, but does not heal wounded internal self- concepts. So you must be ready for all the possible changes that can accompany the physical body change. Do not worry. Usually most changes are positive and desperately needed to allow a better quality of life in health, relationship, public, employment and one's self-worth.

Separation Process

When talking about separation, one must understand the Herd Mentality. People are creatures of habit; they want to fit in with the crowd. During my undergraduate studies, I composed an experiment that strongly suggested that people want to be accepted as one of the group. This was modeled after previous Ash studies that showed people will alter their belief to obtain group conformity. I set up three, different liquids with distinct smells, in unmarked cups. One was water, the other strawberry, and the third apple. Four actors went prior to the test subjects and gave a consistent set of answers to the cups' label. They said out loud for the subjects to hear, "No smell for the water, strawberry for the strawberry and orange for the apple". Many subjects consistently agreed with the actors and labeled the apple as orange. Too many to have happened by chance alone. However, the experiment results where not proven due to many extraneous variables. Give me a break; this was just my undergraduate attempt. The Ash studies were significant and are used to support the theory of the Herd Mentality. People become creatures of habit by eating in the morning on the way to work. Also, when it is 12'o clock let us join the herd in eating lunch. We Americans have forgotten how to listen to our bodies. In the wild, animals eat when they are hungry, not at 12 noon sharp. These are behaviors that need to be eliminated to be successful in weight loss. That is one positive thing about the low carbohydrate/high protein diets. They actually help teach people the difference in mental hunger and physical hunger. They allow a person to usually eat all the meat they want, just limit the carbohydrates. After awhile, you will believe you are hungry but not want to eat any meat. This is a psychological hunger due to the fact that the dieter can eat all the meat they can stand. However, they still desire the taste for other foods. This enables one to truly experience and know the difference between psychological and physiological hunger. Prepare yourself for this separation as there will be social pressure to join the herd. Remember some herds are hazardous to join, for example, the Bebop Comet cult led by Applegate. They all killed themselves thinking they were going with the Bebop Comet. See my point? You must lead yourself instead of depending on others. Get ready to gain support from yourself, because you are going to spend time getting to know yourself. You are going to stick out from the herd. An exercise I challenge my clients to do is to accept a group invitation to lunch. However, I want my clients to just order water when they join the group for lunch. No food. One does not always have to eat just because everyone else does. I want the clients to experience and give feedback on what it was like to change the norm. They all seem to learn by experience that they do not have to eat just because everyone else does. I hope they acquire that they need to eat only when they are physically hungry. Eat for health and fuel, not for social pressure, pleasure, anxiety, depression, boredom or out of just plain old habit.

Awareness

By now you have become aware that you are not happy with your physical appearance or quality of life. In the here and now, you must summon the determination to change. The way you have been living and the decisions that have been made are what have brought about the disappointing consequences. There is good news that will brighten this last statement. You have the power to be unhappy means you also have the power to change and become happy, healthy, fulfilled, and physically appealing.

Most of our problem is the desire for instant self-gratification. Most overweight people know that the negative consequences will happen, yet we still indulge in this self -defeating behavior. We must become aware that there is an instant self- gratification that meets some of our needs. Let us look at binging on three Twinkies. The instant self- gratification needs are as follows:

(1) *Instant sugar high "more energy"*
(2) *Feeling change (Some people even visualize happy thoughts when eating)*
(3) *Satisfy's hunger or stimulates taste receptors and individual pairs this with pleasure stimulus.*

Being aware that these short term gratifiers are being met gives us the opportunity to switch the behavior in order to satisfy these needs. I would encourage you to do other healthy behaviors instead of eating the Twinkies, for example, exercise, eat a protein bar, or call a friend. Replace the behavior with a healthy one, instead of just saying you will not do it. When a person is told not to do something, sometimes he or she carries out the behavior in opposition to what he or she is told not to do. That is exactly why when I hypnotize a client, I empower him to succeed at achieving another behavior that will replace the unwanted one. Changing the behavioral way these short term gratifying needs are met, generates more success in accomplishing the change in the unhealthy behavior. Therefore, change the way to meet the need, change the result.

Awareness within itself is not curative. A sense of direction is needed in adjunct. If you summon a taxicab while at Wal-Mart, the cab driver will ask you where you would like to go. If you answer with, "Well I don't want to go home and I don't want to go to the ballpark", he will get you out of his cab if you do not give him a destination. We focus on what we do not want in life. Clients tell me upon beginning treatment "I don't want to feel depressed". I can not help one achieve what they do not want. Now if they identify within reasonable means what they want, then we can start making a behavioral plan to achieve this goal. A reframing question that would guide my client into taking responsibility is "What would you want to feel like in life?" The client is forced to identify a direction. His response is "I want to feel better than I do now" The client has identified his feelings in the here and now and given latitude for the therapist to assist the client in identifying the direction with the next question of: "Knowing you feel bad now, how would we know when you feel better or what behaviors would you be doing that would identify this change?" Moving the client into a sense of direction is usually needed to produce change. Many people dwell on what they do not want and this stalls them on taking action for change. Actually, it is really a way for a person to avoid responsibility in planning his action, taking action and producing a desired change.

A Worksheet for Behavioral Change

(1) What unhealthy behavior is identifiable?

(2) Identify the short term payoff/gratification/need(s) that are being met?

(3) List at least 6 alternative healthy behaviors that can replace these short term needs.

Carry this list in your pocket and follow-up by committing to doing the alternative behaviors when these needs arise.

List the dates below at the end of each day; these dates are the ones that I <u>did</u> the alternative behaviors.

If you follow this plan, there will be feedback on the days that you are successful. After six weeks, total up the number of days that the alternative behaviors worked. If there are significant more days of the plan working than not, continue the plan. For you mathematicians, I would say success can be measured at 75%. If you are under the 75% rate of success, then it is time to change the alternative behaviors. Apparently, the first behaviors chosen are not meeting the short term needs. Through a process of elimination, you will find what behavior will be successful. This model will hold you self-accountable for achieving change in your behavior.

Management of Eating Behavioral Training Rules (MEBTR)

There are the dreaded rules in every program. The Management of Eating Behavioral Training Rules (MEBTR) will assist in modifying ones eating behaviors while simultaneously strengthening awareness of the habitual eating patterns. One must strictly adhere to the rules for ultimate success. After all, most of us do not expect something for nothing. If this were the case, everyone would have it. The saying is true "You have to work hard for anything that is worth something" At first, the MEBTR may be difficult but with time, adhering to them will become easier.

(Week 1)
  (1) **The first 7 days of the program you are to eat only half of what you normally would eat at a setting.**
  (2) **Replace eating the other half of the plate with a 15 to 30 minute walk.** Remember one gets out of a program what they put into it. This statement should answer the question of, what kind of pace should one be walking? I think it is up to what the individual is capable of applying. The main thing is to get started with the change of behavior, even if the walk is as slow as a snail. **Consistency is the key to success in the program!**
  (The goal of the first week is to shrink the stomach and begin some physical activity.) Remember the amount of food consumed should be equal to the size of your fist balled up. This is about the size of your stomach.
  (3) No matter what, do not fall for the "value trap sell" if eating out at a food place. See this is a major pit fall for many people as we tend to think getting a

good deal on lunch is important. I'm not sure if this
was a belief that we connected in our adult thinking
to the childhood training of cleaning off one's plate.
However this belief was incorporated, the fast food
industry plays this psychological card to the extreme.
See they offer value combo meals with visual displays
that even suggest we save more money by simply
super sizing for a few cents more. Think of the power
of this marketing suggestion. Taking advantage of
childhood eating training and pairing it to getting a
good deal. Wow they may as well ring a bell every
time someone orders food and super sizes it, then
have a worker go out in front ordering counter and
ring that bell while their consumers are viewing the
menu. For those unfamiliar with this scenario, it is
called the conditioned response and discovered by
Ivan Pavlov. A research physiologist that noticed that
the experimental subjects that were dogs would
salivate upon hearing the feeders foot steps. He then
paired a ringing bell with the feeding of the dogs.
Then just rang the bell alone and low and behold the
conditioned response would occur. This was evident
by measuring the increased amount of the dog's
salivation upon hearing just the bell. **Very powerful!**
An environmental stimulus that had stimulated a
physiological response in an animal shows us just
how powerful an environment can be. Keeping this
in mind, I would order one pancake and one strip of
bacon and see that it costs almost as much as ordering
the three pancake combo. This challenged my belief
of getting your moneys worth. However, the price
you pay is your health; as most would eat all three
pancakes and two strips of bacon if ordered and
placed in front of them. Is it worth your health to save
that extra dollar? You really need to be aware that
you are really just viewing artery clogging, fat

21

increasing, and health decreasing servings with a higher probability of ones life expectancy to dramatically shorten. This is my opinion, not research but, I bet that there is a strong positive correlation between heart attacks and people who normally super size their meals on a daily basis. Don't worry the fast food chains will never report this finding even if they have done the research. It would be bad for their business.

(Week 2) (Continue eating as in week one, small portions or half normal servings)

    (1) **When eating, only eat while sitting at a table**. Do not eat in an automobile or while sitting in front of a TV. We eat habitually in front of the TV, at the movies, or while driving. When we do this we are usually eating through unawareness. As stated before, I can remember eating a bucket of popcorn or several slices of pizza, only to think I was hungry 30 minuets later when I found out it was 12 noon. Eating at a designated setting gives us more control over the conscious variables. We are aware we are eating and hopefully not doing it out of habit, but hunger and nourishment.

    (2) **Do not eat for pleasure or as a reward**. Remember our pleasure system pairs rewards or good emotions with our behaviors. This can be destructive to ones mental eating habits. I would take a can of (Meal Replacement Drink) when going to an office party where food is served as a celebration. I would give the rationale that I am on a strict diet for my health. This also allowed me not to have to contribute to funding these eating parties. Also, it is not good to reward yourself with eating whatever you desire. This can lead back to a

bad pattern eating. If you want a reward, purchase something for yourself. After all, it is all about wanting to like yourself, you deserve a reward. At least this way, one can not go wrong with the selection of the gift.

(3) **Do not eat out at fast food restaurants.** Prepare your foods and brown bag it. The mentality is that we want to stop searching for food. I remember driving five miles out of the way just to eat out at a certain restaurant. This would strengthen eating for nourishment and combat the desire of emotional eating.

(4) **If you have a craving for food, go ahead and eat one or two bites**. This will satisfy the craving. Be sure to limit to no more than two bites.

(Week 3) (Continue previous rules)

(1) **Now it is time to consult with a doctor to determine a diet and work out a program for you to start.** I would recommend consulting a doctor that is sensitive to patients who want to become healthy through weight loss. I have had bad experiences with general practitioners who would respond to my questions about weight loss with remarks such as "just push yourself away from the table" This remark was both sarcastic with truthfulness and degrading. I am not advocating getting prescriptions to lose weight. That should be only discussed between you and the doctor and determined by you alone. I personally don't believe in using them due to my approach to weight loss. I believe in changing behavior to get needs met. The way these needs are behaviorally met will be switched. When taking pharmaceuticals it can and

23

usually does assist in weight loss. However, the person does not change their true behavior or internal scripts. This is why they experience the rollercoaster syndrome. The things they changed were chemistry and they learned to adapt to weight loss while on the drug. When the drug is taken away, they experience intense cravings and give in to their old unchanged patterns of eating.

(2) **Focus on one day at a time.** Do not be overcritical of yourself. If you mess up on one meal, that is fine. Do not use that mistake as an excuse to continue messing up. Remember it is not how fast you get somewhere, but it is important to just get there. I would say an ideal goal of weight loss is about 10 pounds a month, about 2 ½ pounds a week is an ideal target.

Mentality

The ideal is to fake it until you make it. Live the life of a person who is on a mission of pursuing health through weight loss. Enjoy and strengthen your motivation as others tell you they notice a difference. Remember you spent a lot of your life overweight and now you are a person concerned with good health and driven to lose weight. Gain more confidence in yourself as you notice your clothes becoming looser in fit. This is an accurate measure of your success. Throw away that scale. The scale may as well be one of those negative people. Your weight changes daily due to water retention. So remove yourself from the negative people who want to bring you down. You are reinventing yourself with healthy eating habits. Remember there is no magic pill for weight loss. You have to ultimately burn more calories than you take in. That means success is a total lifestyle change.

Changes that happen upon success

Upon success of achieving your goals, changes will occur in your life. I have seen many people lose weight and transform themselves into a new lifestyle. Divorces happen when one partner works on self and grows without the other. People change for the better or worse. They tend to view old lifestyles as boring and look for different stimulation. They may blame their spouse or relationship for their weight gain. I sense that weight loss effects one's sexual appeal and desire. That is why divorces are a strong catalyst for weight loss and lifestyle change. You may suffer from financial issues, going wild spending money on clothes or self. You may act as if you are living life and making up for what you feel you missed out on. Career changes happen. People flee towards people who are similar to them. Now that you lost weight, your old friends may become a thing of the past. People usually change their playgrounds, playthings and playmates. So be prepared for many changes that will happen in your life upon your success. I will explain what happens further by addressing happiness.

Meaning and Purpose

Happiness is a product of living one's true meaning and purpose in life. This is of the highest importance in lifestyle change. As mentioned earlier, people are motivated to change in three ways, frustration, health, and existential happenings. This area is what causes so much anger, hurt and pain in a divorce. In a divorce, usually one person wants it and the other does not. In this case, one of the persons started the mental distancing prior to the actual divorce. Now this person files for the divorce and the other person is devastated. Let us say it is the man who did not want the divorce. The man built his whole meaning and purpose around being married to his spouse. He made life and financial decisions based on being with this person. Well she has grown in a different direction and no longer wants to be married. This shatters the man's ideal of meaning and purpose in his life. He feels like he has been living an illusion or lie. Now he is left to pick up the pieces. So he seeks to get his needs met. He usually rebounds. This is where he attempts to replace his spouse with another available female. This is the man's attempt to hang on to the old meaning and purpose. After time, the man starts to see the person is not who he thought her to be (projection). He then leaves because he realizes he was not in love with her and can not believe he even talked about marriage. He was driven unconsciously to obtain that meaning and purpose in life, and then upon acceptance he sees happiness can only come through pursuit of a true meaning and purpose in life.

People who live a mistaken meaning are only going through the motions in life. They are living by habit not life. They go to work, eat some cookies, watch Jay Leno and get up the next day to do the same. A meaning is multiple in nature. People have different meanings. I define a meaning as an identity with a sense of belonging. People get their meaning met by work, church, family or many other entities. Changing your life through weight loss will also affect your meaning and purpose in life. Many people who lose the weight realize they were just going through the motions of life. Their needs of identity and belonging were not being met. The purpose is the drive in our life. My meaning in life is that I am a Dad, counselor, son, etc. and my purpose is to raise my children and help people change. There are different, multiple meanings and different, multiple purposes. Finding ones true meaning is similar to the pursuit of happiness. If you are not enjoying life then look at the area that seems to be keeping you from obtaining a true meaning and purpose. <u>Life is like a video game</u>. There are lots of different games to meet a variety of different peoples' needs. Now that you found the game you like, you put a quarter in and start playing it. You become excited by behaviors of moving a lever or hitting buttons. If I walk up behind the machine and pull the plug from the wall, you can still move the lever and push the buttons (going through the motions) but there is no longer any satisfaction. By pulling the plug I took away all meaning and purpose behind the behavior of moving the lever and pushing the buttons. Life is very similar in that if you're just going through the motions (moving levers, pushing buttons) then you are not going to be happy.

Imagery Guided Change

Imagery is a tool used by many to assist in producing many changes in their lives. Imagery can be a valuable tool to assist with any weight loss program. Studies even show that imagery produces muscle responses when applied. I remember a study of boys shooting free throws. One group practiced shooting free throws for two weeks. The other group went through imagery training of seeing the goal and making the free throw. The other group did nothing. On the first day, all groups were tested on the amount of free throws made. Two of the groups, the one that practiced and the one that relied upon imagery training alone, showed no significant difference in improvement in comparison to one another. Both groups show dramatic improvement over the group that did not practice.

Imagery is more than just seeing oneself perform the action. Although that is one important part, there is a lot more. A person must feel the feelings and act in order to promote the best results. For example, if I wanted to improve my kick boxing techniques, I would imagine myself going through the warm up. I would feel the sweat on my shin as my muscles warm up to the action. I would imagine what it feels like to be an expert and make every kick as sharp, clean, and perfect as possible. I would feel or process the feeling of pride over my accomplishments. I would see myself making every kick, knowing where this would take me in tournaments. I would imagine myself as a champion kick boxer. Attempting to have the same feelings and thoughts as a champion kick boxer, I would practice letting these thoughts and feelings go into my subconscious. Letting go, without obsessing over the thoughts, is key to success. The next practice session or imagery session, I would attempt to reconnect with the earlier imagery work. An exercise I want you to do is make a collage of personal goals in weight loss. Then I want you to put it up in your bedroom where you see it first thing every morning. Making a collage is simple. Just look through old magazines and cut out pictures of where you are now in life, where you want to go, and the means it will take to get there. Most clients cut pictures of people's expressions and interpret them as emotional mindsets. I hope you use some emotional mindsets in your collage building. Making and placing the collage in a well viewed place, will motivate you upon awakening each morning and going to sleep each night.

Utilizing imagery in your weight loss program has many components. First see yourself getting started and feel what it feels like to get started. Really get into it as you feel the pride, determination and motivation to strive for these goals. The next session, see yourself in an eating situation. Imagine combating the impulse to eat unhealthy selections. Feel relief and pumped up about countering that thought and eating a healthy choice selection. Imagine how it feels to overcome these impulses and be in charge of your life. Free yourself from the unhealthy side of self. Imagery will very dependent upon your specific situation and need. Notice I said need. Yes imagery can be one of your alternative healthy behaviors that meet your gratifying need. Imagery must be as realistic as possible to get ultimate results.

Tips to help out

(These are tips that I have gathered by word of mouth. Their accuracies may not be consistent among research. I do believe these tips work or I would not have published them in this book).

   (1) <u>Throw away the scale or just use it once per month to look at progress</u>. Using the fit (tightness or looseness) of one's clothing to measure progress is

much better than weighing on a scale. Scales are abusive since weight can fluctuate daily, even when making progress.

(2) <u>Exercise that is spread throughout the day speeds up metabolism better than all in one hour</u>. I heard this in a health class at A&M. The instructor explained working out 3 times a day for 20 minuets burns more calories than a single one hour session. She explained how the body has a homeostasis that is like a thermostat. By exercising in intervals, the body adapts and sets the metabolism at a higher baseline.

(3) <u>When eating try to cut down all bread portions</u>. When I have a hamburger, I throw the bottom portion of the bun away. This still satisfies my hunger and works for me in reducing size and caloric intake.

(4) <u>Exercise in the morning is more efficient than in the evening</u>. Early in the morning upon awakening, your metabolism is speeding up for the day. Exercise increases this effect. In the evening your metabolism is slowing down and exercise is working against it. Also, when sleeping your body produces growth hormones. Levels are higher in the body during awakening than before bed.

(5) <u>Buy some meal replacement bars for times when food is not available</u>. This will keep you from being tempted at fast food services. I have seen people cheat and eat two of the bars when they were hungry. They rationalized it was better than eating french fries or potato chips. I guess they have a point, but try not to do it.

(6) <u>Imagine that you have no choice but to eat right and exercise</u>. This was one of my favorites. I would pretend that I was poor and couldn't afford

to buy restaurant food. So, I had to eat what I had prepared. (You know I am not sure I was pretending I probably was too poor and this was my justification). I would also pretend that if I didn't exercise, I would go to jail.

(7) <u>Realize it is not a race, but a new way of life</u>. Who cares if your buddy loses more than you? It is about starting a new lifestyle. Too many times, people compare themselves with others progress. A lot of people believe competition is healthy and drives them. I personally believe in acceptance and support, but if you need competition to stay on top of the game, more power to you. For those people who do not, it is not necessary for success.

(8) <u>Reward yourself often for changing yourself</u>. Yes, you deserve it for the work you are doing.

(9) <u>Do not let friends or others influence your program</u>. People get partners in the beginning and do well. However when their partner quits or does not do well it sometimes affects the progress of the partner's partner. You probably should be selfish about your program and do it alone.

(10)   <u>Music seems to help motivate me when doing exercise</u>. Use this to your advantage. Listen to your favorite music.

(11)   <u>If trying to build muscle, there is a magic 30 minute time to eat for optimum results</u>. This thirty minute window is optimal for consuming protein either before or right after weight training. The protein feeds the muscle in development. But remember muscle growth happens during sleep, so get plenty of rest.

Training Taste

People actually train their taste receptors to like certain types of foods. This is the reason that we crave certain foods. We actually condition ourselves on what to like in foods. I learned this when I worked at a video store. The coke machine had a button that was mislabeled. It said Coca-Cola, but pushing it actually sold diet Coca-Cola. Being poor, I was forced every now and then to endure my mistaken vending order. After three weeks I started to crave the Diet Coke. I made the mistake at least once a day. Now by the time I trained myself to the error, I had acquired a taste for Diet Coke. Still twenty years later to this very day, I am still drinking Diet Coke. I have fasted before and believe me food tastes different upon reintroducing it back into your body. Lettuce tastes sweet, cokes taste sugary, and French fries taste greasy. I remember drinking protein drinks and eating those protein bars in the day of the old. Ten years ago, they were down right nasty. All body builders learn to turn off their taste and just drink the stuff. Today the flavors have been greatly improved and they taste pretty good. No they are not going to taste exactly like a Snickers bar, but they have greatly improved from ten years ago. So, if you really give it a try, you can adapt your taste to desire healthier food. You have probably conditioned your taste for fat or sugary foods. I remember I went one month without any sugar at all. After the thirty days, I bought a Coke out of a machine. I was shocked because it was sugary and syrupy. I thought it was gross. If you desire or allow yourself enough time, your body will adapt and adjust to your new healthy eating selections.

The Good, Bad and Ugly of the Different Diets

In my experience as a counselor, I have witnessed people losing weight through various diets. I have seen people on protein diets lose weight. I have seen people on low fat diets lose weight. I have seen people on what I call the Tom Seabourne diet lose weight. All these diets being promoted by nutritionists leaves people confused about choosing the right one. <u>As I mentioned before, the selection is best done between you and your doctor or nutritionist</u>. Please understand my knowledge is just from what I have seen or been told as a counselor. I am not a nutritionist nor am I a doctor of medicine. Below is what I have gathered through experience and is to be taken in that context. Not as medical advice. Once again only you and your doctor know your conditions, so talk with him before starting any new diet.

I actually like and prefer Dr. Seabourne's diet. I will give a very little limited summary. If further information is wanted you can Google his name. He has written a couple of books about fitness and nutrition. Dr. Seabourne's diet is simple, but complicated to adhere to. He proposes that we eat six mini meals. These mini meals consist of one low fat protein with two carbohydrates. One of the carbohydrates needs to be fibrous, and both need to be cooked with little fat and oil. The amount of servings is small, with the protein being the biggest and lean. This diet will increase the metabolism and keep sugar levels balanced. The plus to beginning this diet is usually after eating all six meals one is left with a feeling of fullness. The downside is that one must prepare the meals in advance and this sometimes becomes cumbersome. Another downside is making time to eat six meals in a day. Most employment discourages downtime through eating except during lunch break. One way some people adapt this diet is by utilizing meal replacement bars or drinks. But be careful. All meal replacement bars and drinks are not equal. Some are designed for the high protein group, and they usually have high fat content. For further information read Dr. Seabourne's books. I did use this diet with success. My blood pressure stabilized and so did my sugar count. I had energy and didn't feel deprived of food. The fat loss happened but at a steady slow pace of ten to twenty pounds a month. I incorporated this diet with both forms of exercise (aerobic and resistant). This diet is one I could live on as a permanent lifestyle change.

The next diet is the high protein diet. (Adkins, Protein Power, ect) these diets usually consist of eating all the protein one wants, while limiting the number of carbohydrates. If I recall, the amount of carbs I was allowed to eat during the first three days was 35 to 40. Then I was allowed 90 carbs a day until the amount of weight I needed to lose was gone. Upon obtaining the weight loss goal, I could bump up to 150 to 200 carbs. Unless I started gaining weight, then I would just bump them down. I started out at 285 pounds and went down to 175 pounds. This was accomplished after my marriage of 8 years ended. So I was motivated to lose and work out. These diets usually produce quick results that reinforce the dieter to continue the diet. My results were in four to five months. This diet was successful but with many draw backs. It was very limiting in what you could eat. It sounds good in the beginning eating Bar-B-Q and steak. However, the cravings were intense for carbs. I remember viscously craving orange juice like a mad man. Mood swings came with this diet and frequent urination during the night. I do not think as limiting as this diet is, that I could make it a permanent lifestyle change. The one and most valuable thing that came from this diet is learning the difference between physical hunger and mental hunger. You could eat all the meat you wanted, so you wouldn't go physically hungry. I remember thinking I was hungry and eating some meat only to realize I wasn't hungry. I got so burned out on meat, I just would not eat. The diet produces weight loss through dehydration and burning of fat for fuel. Limiting the carbs causes the body to go into ketosis. This is where the body burns keytones for fuel. It also burns protein and fat. My sugar levels did normalize and my blood pressure did go down on this diet. Even though I don't recommend this type of diet, I believe the South Beach diet is a healthier improvement. The South Beach has separated the good carbs from the bad carbs and isn't so restricted as the previous protein diets. Another similar diet is the Nutri-System Diet. I am hearing positive results about these two recent diets, but I have no experience with either one.

The final and last diet is the traditional low fat diet. People who attempted this one did show results, but very slowly, unless they exercised like crazy. My health instructor talked about this issue. She expressed that the body would interpret the low fat diet as starving. Then the metabolism would slow down as a survival mechanism. I believe this to be true as I have seen many frustrated dieters give up because of the slow results and the feelings of deprivation. The diet meets ones health requirements but is slow in producing results.

All in all, you need to pick a diet with your doctor. There is no magic pill other than exercise. A person must take in fewer calories than they burn physically to produce desired weight loss results. Remember you want to measure your loss by how loosely your clothes began to fit. The reason is many people gain muscle mass which is heavier than fat and get discouraged when weighing.

Which Exercise Routine is Best?

The routine is best fitted to the individual and their needs. That is why we have trainers to design a training regime suited to each individual. I am all for hiring a trainer, unless a person has a limited budget and can not afford one. Trainers are very expensive this day and time. However, a good trainer will listen to you and design a program for you to obtain the desired results. They are taught proper mechanics in exercises, in which, if applied properly, prevents injury. Exercising the proper way also delivers optimum results. It is very easy to do a sit up improperly. One can use their back muscles instead of their stomach muscles. If done incorrectly, effectiveness is greatly reduced. A good trainer does not miss sessions and they watch you doing exercise techniques. I have witnessed some bad trainers that do not watch their clients while exercising. The trainer is being paid to assist you in achieving your goals. They are not paid to do their exercises, socialize, or just stand there while you are exercising. I also want a trainer to motivate me to push myself to constantly improve my exercise performance. Another good point is when people hire a trainer, they are making a personal and financial commitment to obtaining their goal. This behavior tends to lock people into not breaking the commitment. When a trainer is not performing satisfactorily, it is better to let him go and find one that makes you happy. Being happy while exercising is beneficial in keeping you focused and motivated. This is why I would have a 'cancellation for any reason' clause in any contract made with a trainer. Any respectable trainer would allow such an item in their contract, as they know that they cannot help everyone. Personalities clash and many other things can intervene in a trainer-client relationship. Therefore, be extremely careful before signing any contract with a fitness trainer. Be sure everything that is promised is in writing. My advice is not to be construed as legal advice. Only your attorney can give you legal advice, so I always recommend consulting with your attorney before accepting any legal contractual relationship. Utmost, **BE CAREFUL!**

Going at It Alone Without a Trainer

In today's society, not all of us are able to afford a trainer. There are different types of exercise regimes that produce different results, and different ways to gain knowledge about exercising affordably. I will share my secrets to exercising on a budget share the tips I have obtained about exercising throughout my experience as a graduate health/fitness student, karate student, body builder in the public gyms and sports training (football, baseball, kick boxer, soccer, distance track runner and speed skater).

One excellent way to get training is at the local community college. One can take physical activity courses as continuing education. Most community colleges offer non-credit courses available to the public. This allows the college to give access to the public that do not have the qualifications to enroll in college or to those who just want to enhance their skills without seeking a degree. The advantage is that you get access to college services such as professional instructors, and exercise facilities. The best part is the price which is usually much less than the regular tuition for a one hour credit course. Think about that. What a deal. You get a professional instructor's assistance and up to 4 months of access to the college's exercise facility. Another bonus is that by being enrolled, you have access to the college's library where you can find any information needed about exercise programs. The college libraries have abundance of physical fitness books and videos. If they do not have what you are looking for, then they can order it through other college libraries. This is the best way to get assistance with your weight loss program without a trainer.

Joining a health club costs money and usually involves signing a binding long-term contract. Be careful upon joining the clubs. Usually most clubs will give a one week, free membership so that an individual can try out their facility. If not, then it is better to pay a few times to see what the facility and staff are like. The clubs have classes usually at an extra charge. Some offer personal staff trainers to motivate new members to join. If so, be sure to get it writing and when it will happen. It would, also, be good to know beforehand exactly what this person's duties will be. Will he just assist when asked, will he watch only you, and will he design a personal plan just for you? Do not expect too much from a trainer provided by the club. This is usually just a sales draw to get you to join the club. They usually only help with exercise techniques and have so many other duties, they are seldom available. Generally, the free trainer is a good source to get tips from and some prewritten exercise regimes, but do not expect the same services as hiring a personal one. Joining a club needs to be thought out. The commitment strengthens the motivation to adhere to the exercise program. Be sure to visit all nearby clubs before deciding which one to join. Do not join out of high pressure sales or impulse. Shop around and be sure to get the best deal for the money.

There are additional methods to obtain physical fitness education without hiring a trainer. Thousands of fitness books and videos are available to the public through local libraries and video store rent some under special interest sections. I have seen some excellent routines and lessons for free on the fitness channels. Looking for equipment takes patience, but start with a garage sale. I have never gone to a garage sale that did not have either exercise equipment or books available. I have gotten excellent bargains at garage sales. Remember if you can not afford too much, the best investment is in a good pair of running shoes.

My Knowledge on Exercise Programs

There are many different ways to exercise, especially to tone up and shrink unwanted fat cells. I have tried both aerobics and resistance training programs. A combination of both is best for toning up and weight loss. I personally prefer a type of resistance called power sets. This exercise is resistance based, but aerobic methods are mixed into the regime and last about forty-five minutes to an hour. They have produced great results for me throughout the past. Whichever program you use, there are things that need to be incorporated into any regime.

First, stretching the muscles in a five minute warm-up can prevent injuries. I begin with basic stretches learned in physical education during my school years, such as the hurdler, toe touches, and squats. When stretching, it is important not to bounce the muscles. One must actually pull the muscle while relaxing it to gain flexibility. Once at the end of a stretch, hold it to the count of five and feel the burn. It is important to stretch all muscles in the body, even if the exercise does not utilize that certain muscle.

Second is the warm up phase. This is where one does ten minutes of aerobic exercises that get the blood flowing and heart pumping. This conditions the body to gradually get into a high, heart beating pulse. These exercises are also designed to loosen the muscles. The exercises are toe touches, jumping jacks, rocking chair, arm circles, high knees and pushups. Do not just confine yourself to these exercises. There are many that do the trick. Just be sure to target the whole range of muscles. Ten minuets is enough time to loosen up and get the heart pumping in preparation for more intense workout. These two prior workout components are extremely important for non- injury performance.

Third, the actual best workout regime is a mixture of both aerobic and resistance training. The resistance training will increase muscle mass. Do not worry. It is very doubtful you are going to look like Arnold Schwarzenegger or any of those gross body builders. Obtaining those types of results takes excessive training, strict diet and lots of time. Most people even if they wanted too, would have difficulty achieving this type of body. I always get a laugh at females who refuse to lift weights because of fear of this type of growth. The routine is do resistance training three days a week and aerobic two days a week. One needs at least one day a week rest, so go ahead and rest the whole weekend. Unless you are an overachiever, then add a day of aerobic or weight strength training. A typical schedule would be:

> *Monday- work the chest and arms*
> *Tuesday- aerobic jogging of at least forty-five minutes, if not an hour. Wednesday –work the back and shoulders*
> *Thursday- jump rope for at least forty-five minutes to an hour*
> *Friday-exercise the legs and stomach*

For the overachievers, Saturdays would be whole body exercises such as squats, power clings and dead lifts, or swimming laps in a pool. If you prefer aerobics then a day of karate, bicycling, volleyball or any other aerobic activity you enjoy. By following this plan, you get an equal blend of fat reducing exercises.

People ask me "how does resistance training assist with weight loss"? It is true that muscle mass is heavier than fat and it is possible that a person gaining muscle may not lose weight, but could even gain weight. The weight is not important. What is important is shrinking the fat cells. Resistance training increases the muscle mass which speeds up the metabolism. The bigger the muscles, the more energy is required so your body can either take in more calories or just let the fat cells burn for energy. This is a double bonus, getting tone and shrinking fat cells.

Finally, one has to do a cool down period of at least ten minuets to bring the body back down to normal homeostasis state. This is an excellent time to listen to a motivational hypnotic CD. There are many ways to cool down. I prefer to walk until my heart rate goes back to normal. If you do not have a monitor, then it is when you feel comfortable enough to talk without gasping for air. Usually, ten minutes is sufficient however, I like to do more. This is a peaceful time and excellent trance inducing period. I listen to music during exercising and the hypnotic trance during the cool down phase.

Life changes from a counselors view

The process of change in a person is subjective and interpreted differently by the many driven theories. Year long arguments over Nature vs. Nurture still plague today's sciences. Throughout my career I have viewed evidence of both traits affecting many clients' process of change. Each client exhibits unique strengths and weaknesses. There is no one shoe program that will fit all clients. After all there is no such medicine that will cure mental illness. The medicines' of today have advanced, but still only treat the symptoms without curing the illness. That is what makes weight loss change unique due to the changes occurring on many different levels. Changes must occur in the belief system, motivational system, reward system behavioral system, social system, family system and the physiological system. Even though change in weight loss affects multiple systems; it all begins in one's own awareness.

Awareness is the first factor necessary for free will change to occur. Without awareness no free will change will occur. I have identified three factors that motivate a person to seek change. These catalyst factors are frustration, comfort and Existential Events. They are explained by the following:

(1) <u>Frustration</u> Clients become so sick and tired of living the lifestyle in the manner that they have been living; through internal drives of frustration they seek a life change. This is my theory of the clients needs not being met in daily life. They tend to be going through the motions of life either in chaos or dissatisfaction. Sometimes they even experience a fear of change due to their self imposed comfort zone. Then they become aware

of self inflicted pent up feelings of frustration surfacing and seek change through a fueled motivational driven purpose of seeking new meaning in their lives.

(2) <u>Mental Healthiness</u> The client seems motivated by healthiness to change. The client is living their meaning and purpose, but has the awareness to continue to grow and develop the healthiness of the internal self. Change is necessary to continue living as we know that physiological cessation of change is death. The mental self changes through growth and development is what I perceive as developing spirituality. Being in tune within ones meaning and purpose with continued self awareness in meaningful growth in relationship to self, others and the universe.

(3) <u>An Existential Event/Act of God</u> This is an uncontrollable catalyst that can be identified as a powerful euphoric event in ones life that affects his or her meaning and purpose. A near death experience, death of a loved one or a spiritual awakening that influences are powerful and impact a person to change his or her ways are examples of the Existential Event.

I utilize a formula for Free Will change that has been influenced by multiple theories. The formula contains the following steps:

(1) <u>Awareness</u> One must become aware that a problem exist and accept that he/she has the responsibility to alter self in relation to the problem. A trap of believing in controlling the situation haunts many people in addressing their problems. The thinking error is my behavior controls the situation. Many of my clients end up having to attend Anger Management Class due to their behavior reacting

from this faulty internal belief. They ended up breaking a law in pursuing a partner who no longer wished to be their partner. I have asked many clients "what magical thinking were you thinking?" Did your thinking go "if I harass him or her long enough, then they will eventually come to their senses and say "You were right, I love you and should of never left" The error in thinking is easily compared to a person who believes he or she can just walk out in the pouring rain and command the rain to stop. The logical thinking would be to use adjustment reaction of opening an umbrella. My point is that one cannot control situations, what has happened, or other people. They do have control over self perception and their adjustment reaction to the situation.

(2) Insight/Direction   The client must have the ability to know what he wants to change. Most clients tell me they don't want to feel bad or depressed. I confront them in that I cannot help them with what they don't want. I have them identify what they do want. I do this through many techniques. For instance, my response would have been the question of "What would you life be like if you were happy"? This assists the client in identifying the parts of his life that he could change to achieve happiness. This develops goals with a sense of direction for the client to pursue. The client must identify and know what direction is needed for his desired change.

(3) Planning   Once the client identifies what he or she wants to accomplish, then he or she can gather all information to form a plan of change. Although plans don't always work; the client experiencing independence through self empowerment of attempting to resolve their own issues results in therapeutic growth. Clients must learn to accept failure as an inspiration to further pursue solutions, not just give up. This strengthens the clients evaluation and coping

skills, as several attempts with no success may force the client to reevaluate his or her goals. Take for instances a forty year old out of work actor. Years of rejections for major movie parts may force him or her to accept that acting may just become a hobby and not their profession. The old saying of "if one or two people call you an elephant, don't worry. Now if numerous more on a consistent basis call you an elephant, then its time to buy some peanuts" Design a plan that utilizes strengths and hope that the strengths make up for the weaknesses.

(4) <u>Motivation</u>   Motivation is similar to washing ones hands. Do it daily until it becomes a natural habit. Motivation consists of two catalysts: Internal vs. External. When I worked in an In-Patient treatment center I noticed a lot of the developmentally delayed children would not always groom their hair. So I extrinsically rewarded them for combing their hair. Using the shaping model requires a gradual backing off of the external reward. This promotes the external reward to develop as an internal reward. The goal is for the child to desire grooming their hair because it makes them look good and they desire to look good and groomed. Not because they get rewarded for doing it. External is a stronger reward in the short term race. Internal is stronger in the long term race. Lifestyle change through weight loss is similar. One needs to make a true lifestyle intrinsic eating behavioral change.

Success stems in a positive correlation of a combination of the clients' motivation, awareness, willingness, meaning and purpose direction and readiness to change. The above information can be used as is or even modified for each and every client's specific needs. Remember success isn't always the trait we are hoping will improve when measuring. Sometimes success comes in other forms and within time we become aware of it. The old saying sums this up "Thank God for unanswered prayers".

Summing It All Up

Nothing is easy in life; one has to strive for success. At the end of the tunnel is light. It is easier to maintain a body that is in shape, than getting one into shape. Every time you want to quit, you must gain courage from the inner self. People do not realize how well we have it here in America. We do fall prey to the comfortable lifestyle. This is where we just go through the motions in life. Unaware we substitute emotional needs through unhealthy habitual behaviors. When this happens we must step out of the comfort zone in order to be happy and healthy. Change is necessary throughout life. Otherwise, we quit changing physically which we call death. Sometimes we must experience a metaphoric death in the way we exist to become alive again. Let us live for today and be happy, healthy and prosperous. Life is short and sweet; do not ferment it through complaining, whining, blaming or making excuses. Live it as though tomorrow is your last and enjoy the gift that God has given you.

About the Author

Joseph D. Hayes received his Masters of Science in Community Counseling from Texas A&M Commerce in 1997. He has worked nine years as a Licensed Professional Counselor in the State of Texas. During this time he has developed multiple expertises in working with clients. His work experience began in an out-patient substance abuse treatment facility. There he received vast experience in working with addiction and other mental issues with both court and volunteer cliental. This experience was valuable to Mr. Hayes in that he acquired many skills that laid the foundation of his counseling practice today. There he experienced a unique program called Intensive Intervention Diverse Program. This was a program that he was allowed to assist in group leadership, alternative activities, long term treatment vs. short term treatment therapies, alternative group techniques and individual counseling treatment of cliental. Working with this population allowed Mr. Hayes to treat many different areas of the human psyche under the supervision of Curt Pitton MA. Mr. Hayes has also has had the privilege of serving as a counselor in an In-Patient hospital for children with mental illness. During this work experience, Mr. Hayes has performed a lot of services through his Private Practice. Today he still works performing services through his full time private practice. He also has a self help website at www.coolanger .com where he teaches online anger management. He takes pride in his accomplishments, especially considering that for a couple of years he was a high school drop out. Upon getting his life back on track, he went back to school to graduate with a high school diploma at the age of twenty. Through all that he has accomplished, he expresses his most important job is raising and living with his two children as a single father. He holds many certifications, including National Certified Counselor (NCC), Anger and Depression Specialist, and is certified by the American Board of Hypnotherapy as a Registered Hypnotherapist. If you want to contact Mr. Hayes for services, you can email him through his website at www.coolanger.com. Mr. Hayes would like to leave you with a part of his self through a poem he has written through out his life.

Abandonment

Resentment bound by chains
Keeps me captive with the pain
Born alone, the same as the day I will die
Reality I lived, was nothing but a lie

I'm no fool, but I'm lost
Broken promises, leaves me suffering the cost
Life is merely a series of doors
Opening and closing, as one flees down the corridors
One must not be leery
Even though, this change is scary

The fantasy of opening the door that was shut
Plays on ones sanity with illusions running amuck
Thanatos drives reflected in the mirror
The relationship shattered, Cessation more clearer

Giving the persons Gestalt, can only be a sin
A theme ravages with no true win
She is gone, I could of never done the same
Fore I am human in this life, where people play cruel games

Joseph Hayes

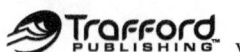 www.trafford.com

North America & international
toll-free: 1 888 232 4444 (USA & Canada)
phone: 250 383 6864 ♦ fax: 250 383 6804 ♦ email: info@trafford.com

The United Kingdom & Europe
phone: +44 (0)1865 722 113 ♦ local rate: 0845 230 9601
facsimile: +44 (0)1865 722 868 ♦ email: info.uk@trafford.com

10 9 8 7 6 5 4 3 2 1

www.ingramcontent.com/pod-product-compliance
Lightning Source LLC
Chambersburg PA
CBHW061225280526
45784CB00006B/2633